Water Aerobics for seniors

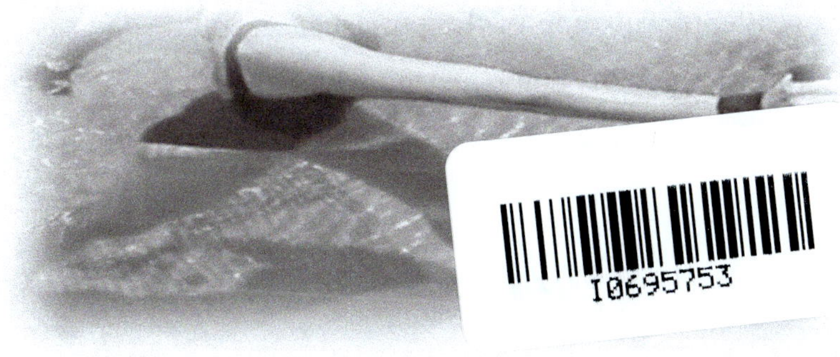

Low impact workout to stay fit and healthy with Pictures

Robert M. Peery

TABLE OF CONTENT

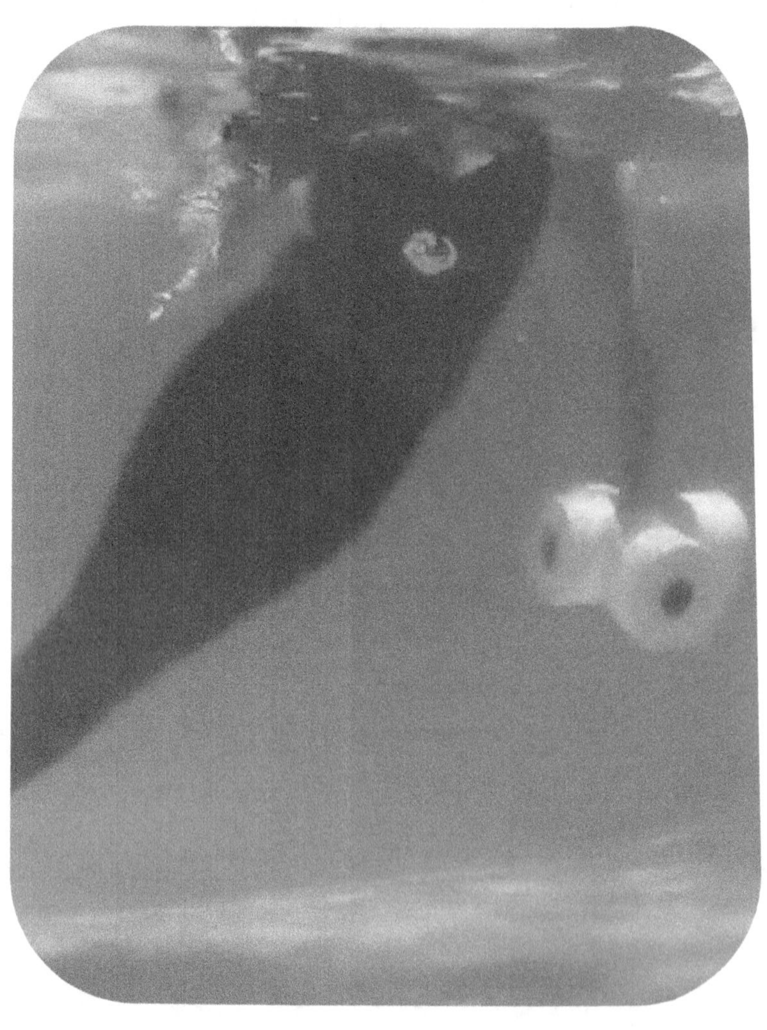

INTRODUCTION

Welcome to the invigorating world of "Water Aerobics for seniors: low impact workout to stay fit and healthy as you age " This book is dedicated to our beloved senior citizens who wish to maintain an active and healthy lifestyle while enjoying the benefits of exercising in the soothing embrace of water.

Water aerobics is a low-impact exercise that offers numerous advantages for seniors, especially for those dealing with joint pain, arthritis, or mobility challenges. The buoyancy of water reduces the impact on joints, making it a safe and gentle exercise option. Moreover, the water's resistance adds an element of strength training, enhancing muscle tone and overall fitness.

Picture Mary, a sprightly 72-year-old grandmother who suffered from chronic back pain and found it difficult to stay active. Struggling with limited mobility, she often felt isolated and disconnected from her community. However, her life took a joyous turn when she joined a local water aerobics class specifically designed for seniors. As the water cradled her body, she discovered newfound freedom and liberation from her pain. Her social circle expanded, and she formed strong bonds with her fellow aqua-aerobic enthusiasts. Mary's story is just one of the many inspiring examples that demonstrate how water aerobics can rejuvenate the spirit and reignite a zest for life in seniors.

Throughout the pages of this book, we will showcase the science-backed benefits of water aerobics for seniors. We will delve into the physiological aspects, exploring how this aquatic exercise improves cardiovascular health, strengthens muscles, and enhances flexibility. Additionally, we will discuss the mental health aspects, exploring how water aerobics can reduce stress, improve mood, and boost cognitive function.

Whether you are looking to embrace a new form of exercise, seeking relief from physical discomfort, or longing to expand your social circle, "Water Aerobics for Seniors" promises to be a valuable resource. Join us as we celebrate the beauty of life in the golden years and dive into the refreshing world of water aerobics. Let's take this plunge together and discover the transformative power of this joyful and revitalizing exercise.

What is Water Aerobics?

Water aerobics is a low-impact aerobic exercise that is performed in water. It is an excellent method for getting an entire-body workout without overtaxing your joints. The buoyancy of the water helps to support your weight, so you can move more freely and easily. This makes water aerobics a good choice for people of all fitness levels, including those with arthritis, back pain, or other health conditions.

Water aerobics workouts typically involve a variety of exercises, such as:

- Water walking
- Aqua jogging
- Arm circles
- Leg lifts
- Jumping jacks
- Squats
- Crunches
- Planks

You can also use water weights, kickboards, and other pool equipment to make your workout more challenging.

In addition to being a great way to get in shape, water aerobics also has a number of other benefits, including:

- Weight loss
- Improved cardiovascular health
- Increased flexibility
- Reduced stress
- Improved mood
- Pain relief

If you're looking for a fun and low-impact way to get a great workout, water aerobics is a great option. There are many different water aerobics classes available, so you can find one that fits your fitness level and interests.

The Benefits of Water Aerobics for Seniors

Here are some of the specific benefits of water aerobics for seniors:

> It is a low-impact activity, therefore it is gentle on the joints. This is important for seniors who may have arthritis or other joint problems.

> It is a fantastic method for enhancing cardiovascular health. Water aerobics can help to increase heart rate and circulation, which can help to reduce the risk of heart disease and stroke.

> Flexibility and range of motion can be enhanced. This is important for seniors who may be starting to experience stiffness in their joints.

> It can help to reduce stress and improve mood. The buoyancy of the water can help to create a feeling of weightlessness, which can be very relaxing.

> It is a fun and social activity. Many water aerobics classes are held in group settings, which can be a great way to meet new people and make friends.

If you are a senior who is looking for a fun and healthy way to stay active, water aerobics is a great option. There are many different water aerobics classes available, so you can find one that fits your fitness level and interests.

Getting Started with Water Aerobics

Here are the steps to take in starting water aerobics:

1. Talk to your doctor. Before starting any new exercise program, it is important to talk to your doctor,

especially if you have any health conditions. Your doctor can help you determine if water aerobics is right for you and can give you any specific instructions or precautions.

2. Find a class that is right for you. There are many different water aerobics classes available, so take some time to find one that is right for your fitness level and interests. Some classes are designed for beginners, while others are more challenging. You may also want to find a class that is held in a pool that is heated, as this can be more comfortable for seniors.

3. Get the right gear. You must dress comfortably so that you may move about easily. You may also want to wear water shoes or aqua socks to protect your feet from the pool floor.

4. Start slowly. Even if you are in good shape, it is important to start slowly with water aerobics. The buoyancy of the water can make it easy to overdo it, so take your time and gradually increase the intensity of your workouts.

5. Listen to your body. Stop exercising and take a break if you experience any pain. Water aerobics should be fun and enjoyable, so don't push yourself too hard.

6. Have fun! Water aerobics is a great way to stay active and have fun. So relax, enjoy the water, and let the buoyancy of the water help you get a great workout.

7. Warm up before you start. This will lower your risk of injury and help your body get ready for exercise.

8. Cool down after you finish. This will help your body to recover from exercise and prevent muscle soreness.

9. Drink plenty of water. Water aerobics can be dehydrating, so it is important to drink plenty of fluids before, during, and after your workout.

10. Take breaks if you need them If you need a break, you shouldn't feel guilty about taking one. Listen to your body and take a break when you need it.

Equipment Need for Water Aerobics

Kickboard: A kickboard is a foam board that you can use to help you float and support your upper body while you work your legs.

Water weights: Water weights are weighted objects that you can use to add resistance to your exercises. They come in a variety of sizes and weights, so you can find the right ones for your fitness level.

Pull buoy: A pull buoy is a foam tube that you can place between your thighs to help you float and support your legs while you work your arms.

Floaties: Floaties are small, inflatable devices that you can use to help you float and support your body weight. They are a good option for people who are new to water aerobics or who have difficulty staying afloat.

Goggles: Goggles are a good idea if you wear contacts or if you have sensitive eyes. They will help to protect your eyes from the chlorine in the pool and from the water itself.

Swim cap: A swim cap is not essential, but it can help to keep your hair out of your face and prevent it from getting wet.

In addition to these essential pieces of equipment, there are a number of other accessories that you may want to consider, such as:

Water shoes: Water shoes can help to protect your feet from the pool floor and from sharp objects.

Towel: A towel is a must-have for drying off after your workout.

Water bottle: A water bottle is essential for staying hydrated during your workout.

Snacks: If you are working out for an extended period of time, you may want to bring some snacks with you to keep your energy levels up.

These are just a few of the equipment you need for water aerobics. With the right gear, you can get a great workout and have fun in the water.

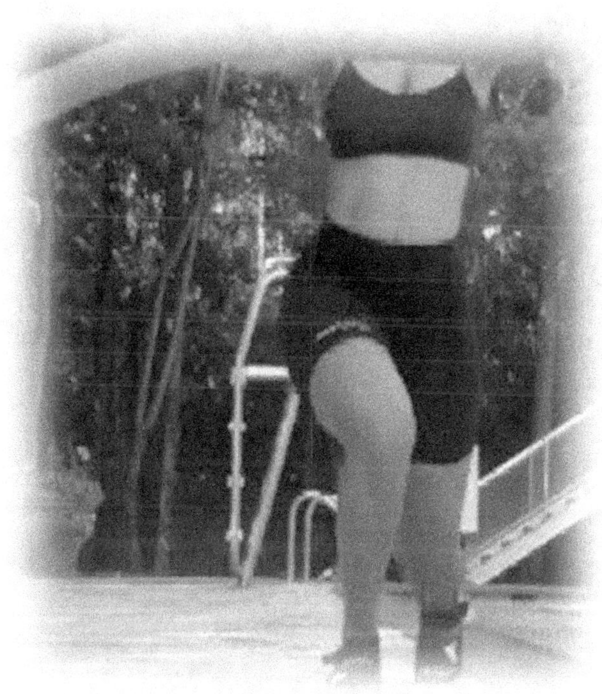

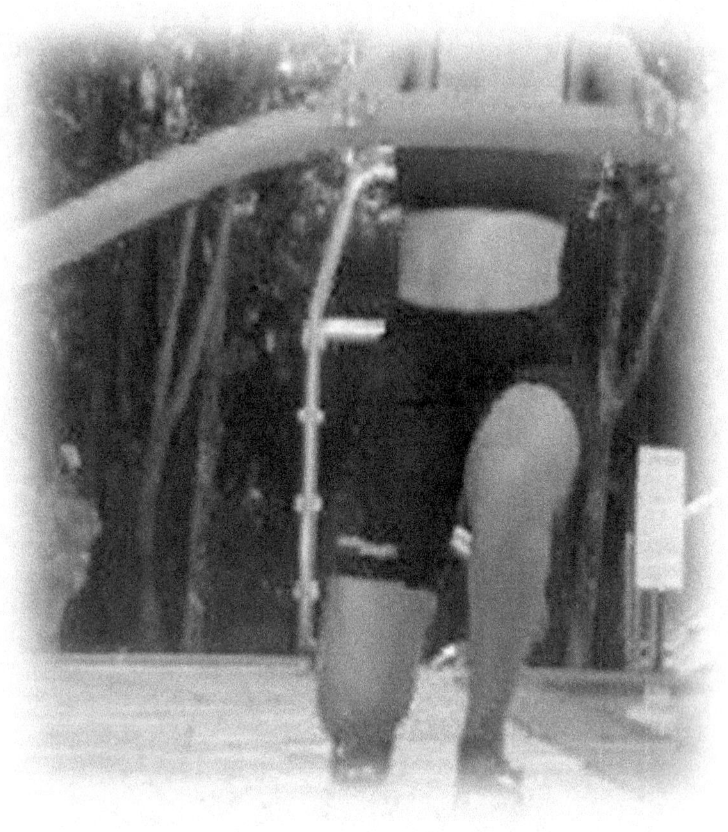

CHAPTER 1: WARM-UP EXERCISES

Here are some of the warm-up exercises that are commonly used in water aerobics:

Arm Circles

This is a fantastic method to warm up your upper body and shoulders. Start by standing in waist-deep water and making broad, forward- and backward-moving circles with your arms. This exercise can also be performed with the arms raised overhead.

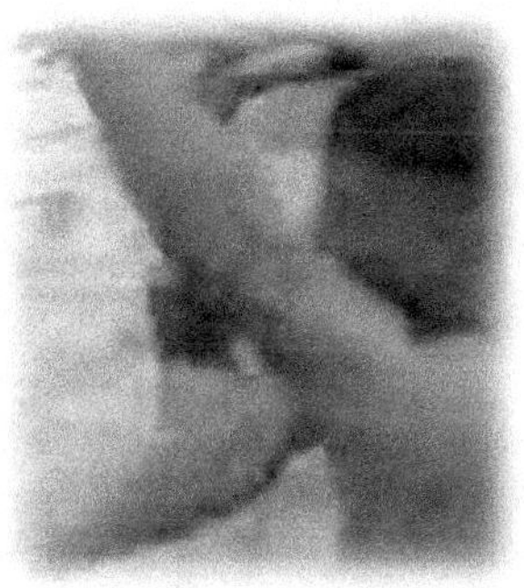

Leg Swings

Your lower body will warm up well if you do this. Swing your legs back and forth while standing in waist-deep water with your knees slightly bent. This exercise can also be performed with your legs extended to the sides.

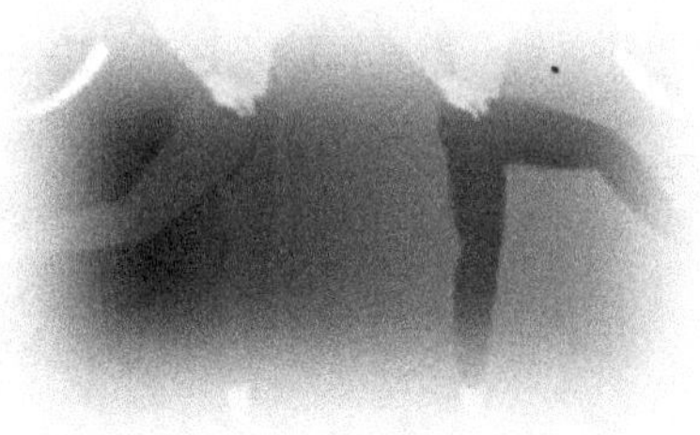

Jumping Jacks

This traditional warm-up exercise is excellent for raising your heart rate. Jump up while standing in waist-deep water by bringing your legs together and raising your arms above your head.

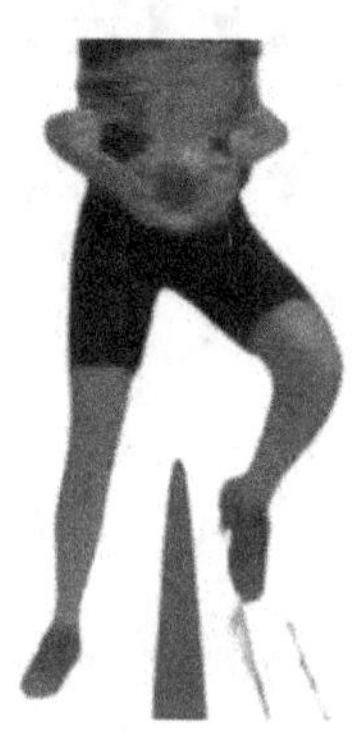

High Knees

Your legs and heart will feel much better after doing this. Standing in the water up to your waist, raise your knees to your chest.

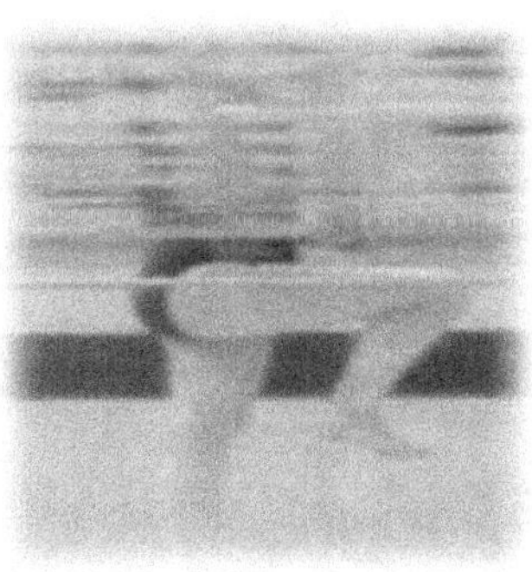

Butt Kicks

You may warm up your glutes and hamstrings by doing this. Kick your heels back till they reach your buttocks while standing in water that is waist deep.

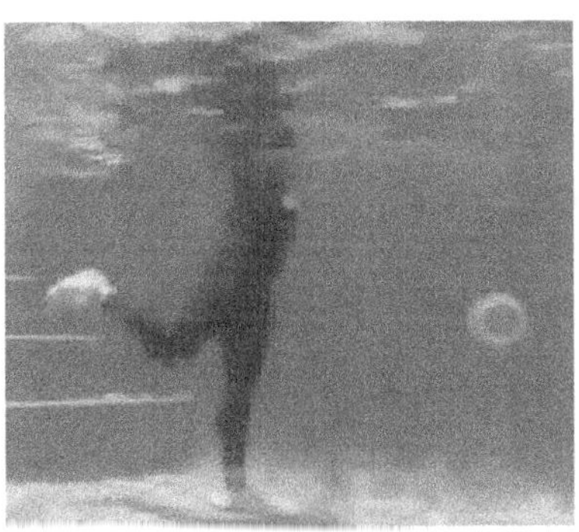

Arm Waves

This is a fantastic method to warm up your upper body and shoulders. Standing in the water with your elbows slightly bent, wave your arms in a side-to-side motion.

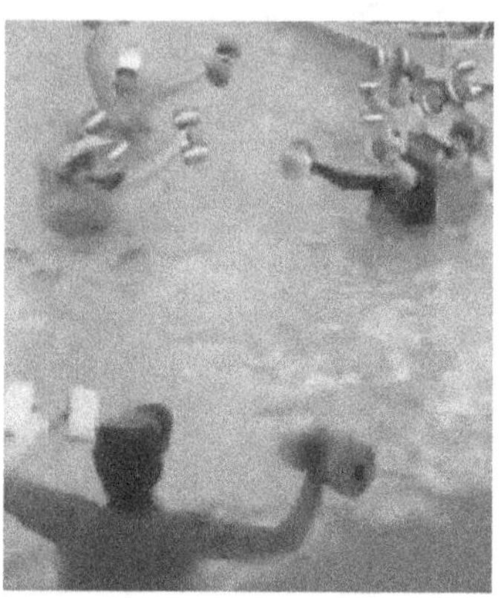

Shoulder Rolls

Warming up your shoulders and upper back by performing shoulder rolls is an excellent idea. Roll your shoulders forward and backward while standing in waist-deep water with your arms at your sides.

Neck Rotations

Warming up your neck and upper back in this manner is beneficial. Standing in the water up to your waist, slowly turn your head to the right, then to the left.

CHAPTER 2: WATER AEROBIC EXERCISES

Aqua Jogging

This is a fantastic technique to exercise your heart while swimming. Standing in water up to your waist, begin jogging stationary. To aid in floating, you can perform this exercise while using a kickboard.

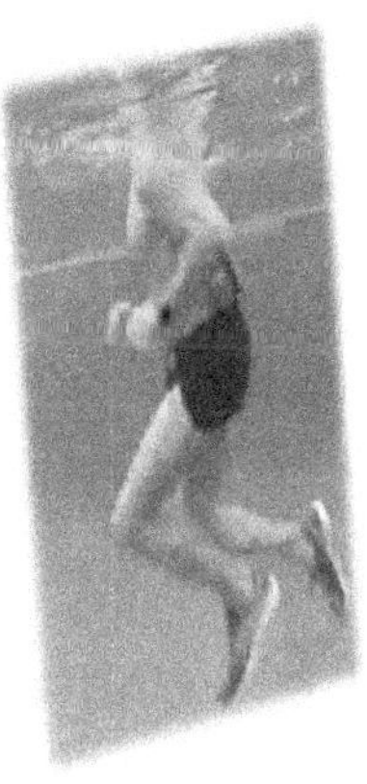

Water Walking

A low-impact exercise in the water is water walking. Similar to walking, but with less strain on your joints thanks to the buoyancy of the water. Standing in water that is at least waist deep, begin water walking by moving forward. To help you stay in place throughout this exercise, you can also use a water treadmill.

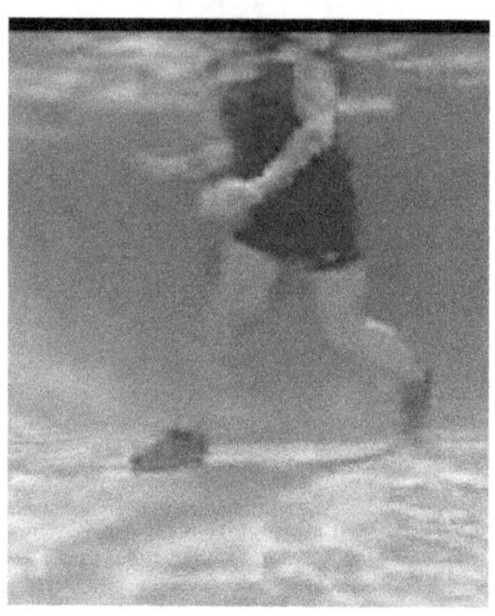

Arm Curls

Biceps can be effectively worked out using arm curls. Start by standing in waist-deep water with a pair of water weights in your hands and perform arm curls there. Curl the weights up towards your shoulders while bending your elbows.

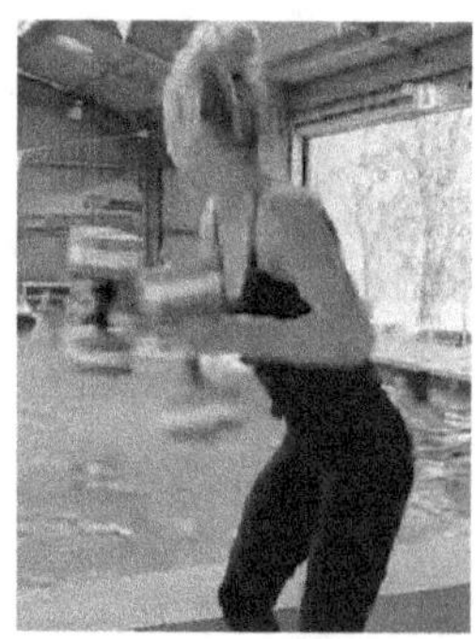
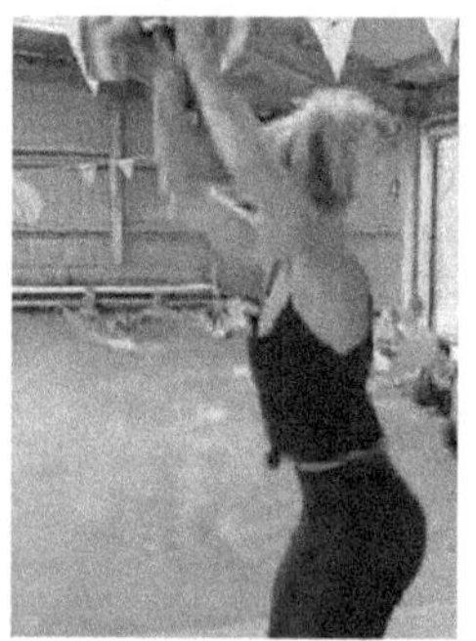

Standing Water Push-ups

Push-ups while standing in water are a fantastic exercise for your chest and triceps. Start by standing in waist-deep water with your hands on the pool's edge to perform standing water push-ups. When your chest meets the water, bend your elbows and squat down.

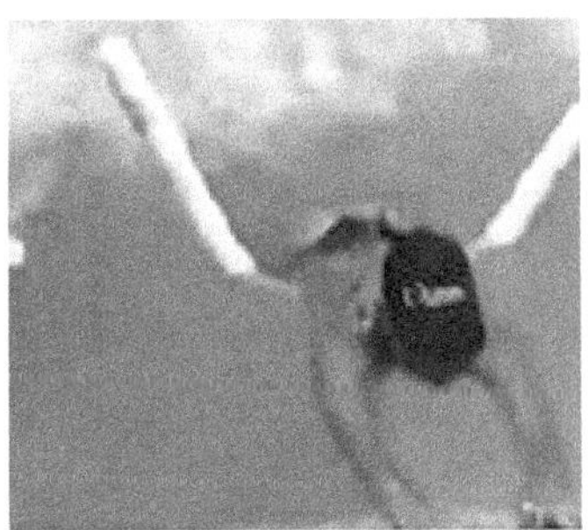

Calf Raises

Your calves will benefit greatly from calf raises. Start by standing in waist-deep water with your weight on your heels to perform calf lifts in the water. Lift your heels as high as you can off the ground.

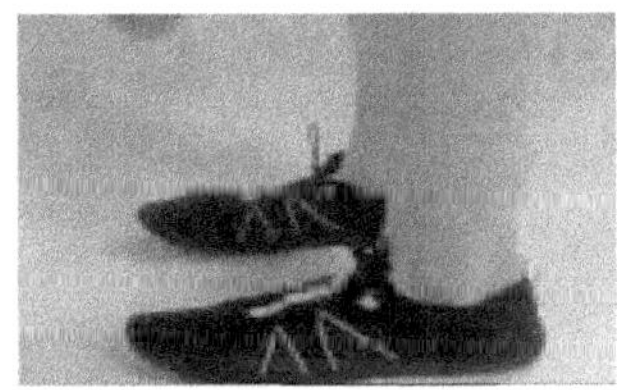 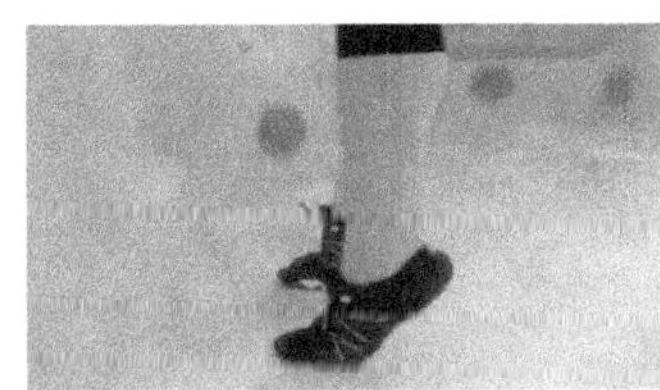

Flutter Kicks

The lower body can be effectively worked with flutter kicks. Start with floating on your back in waist-deep water to perform flutter kicks there. Kick your feet up and down in a fluttering motion while bending your knees.

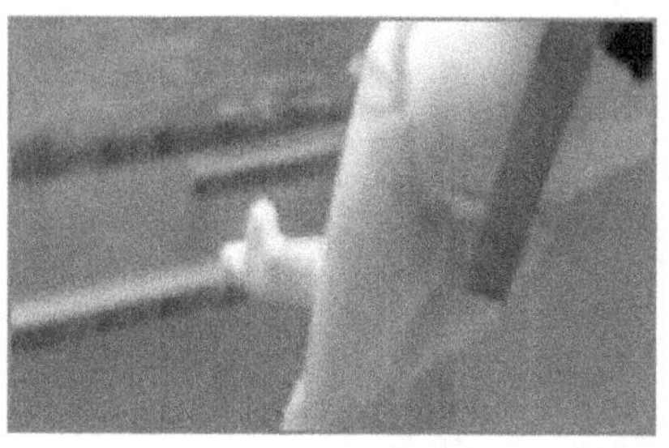 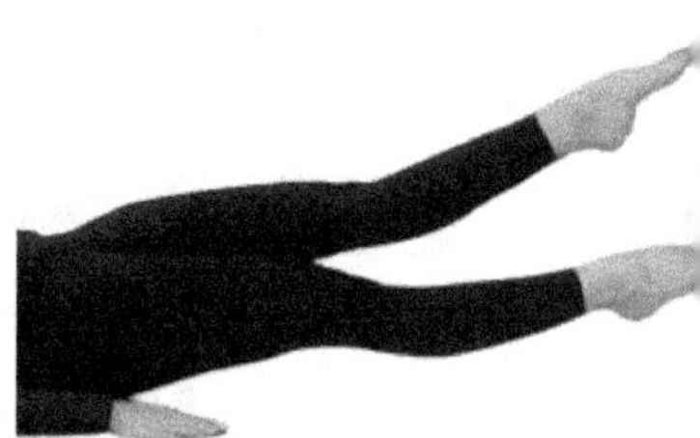

Side Leg Lifts

A wonderful exercise for your obliques is a side leg lift. Float on your back in waist-deep water to begin side leg raises in the water. As high as you can, lift one leg out of the water while bending both knees.

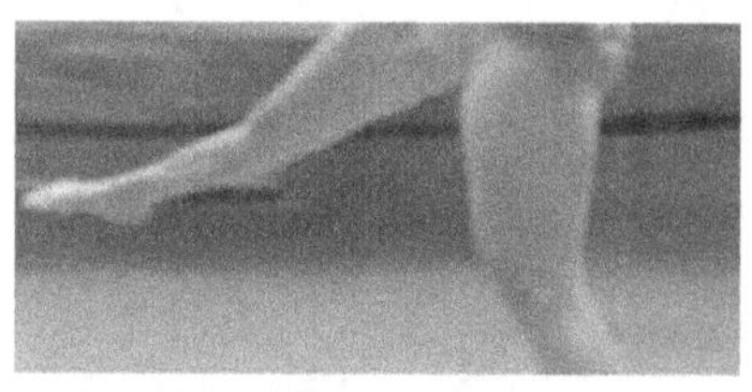

Jumping "Rope"

Jumping rope is a great way to get a cardio workout in the water. To do jumping rope in water, start by standing in waist-deep water and start jumping rope. You can also do this exercise with a kickboard to help you float.

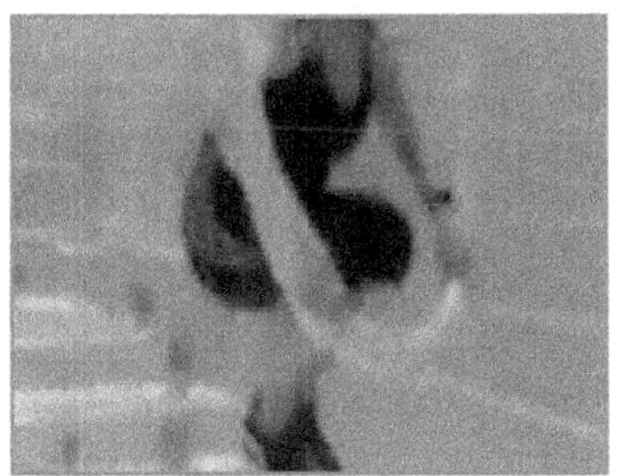 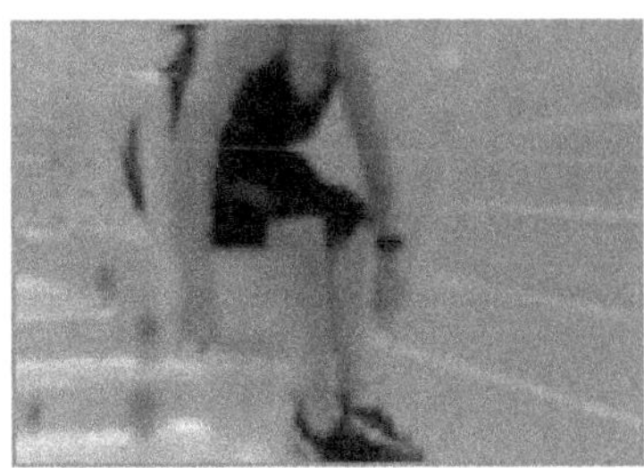

Water Crunches

Work your abs well with water crunches. Float on your back in waist-deep water to begin performing water crunches. Curl your body up as though performing a crunch by bringing your knees up to your chest.

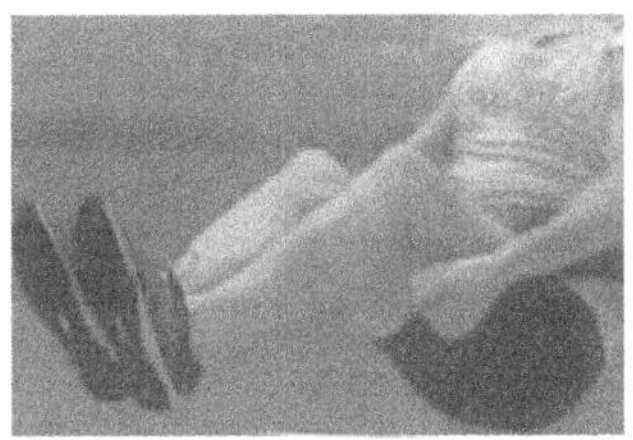

Water Plank

The water plank is a fantastic exercise for your core. Start by floating on your stomach in waist-deep water to perform the water plank. Maintain a straight line from your head to your heels while supporting yourself on your forearms.

This is a popular core-strengthening exercise that involves holding a position that resembles the top of a push-up is known as the standard plank. To carry out a simple plank exercise:

Start by assuming the push-up posture, placing your palms flat on the noodle.

Your feet should be hip-width apart, and your body should be in a straight line from your head to your heels.

Draw your navel toward your spine to activate your core muscles.

Avoid any sagging or arching in your back and keep it flat.

Hold this position for as long as you can while maintaining perfect form; when you first start, aim for at least 20 to 30 second

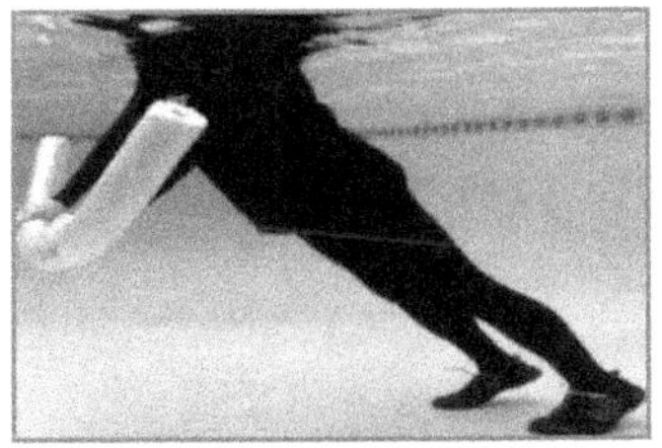
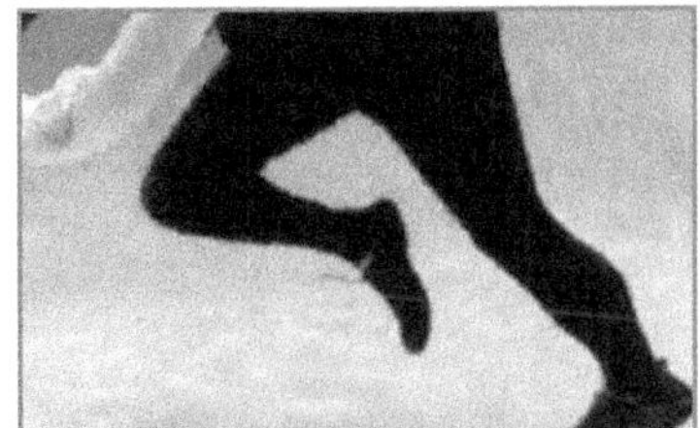

Aqua aerobics with weights

This is a fantastic method to add resistance to your training. Start by swinging your legs or performing arm circles while holding a pair of water weights in your hands. This exercise can be combined with a number of other exercises.

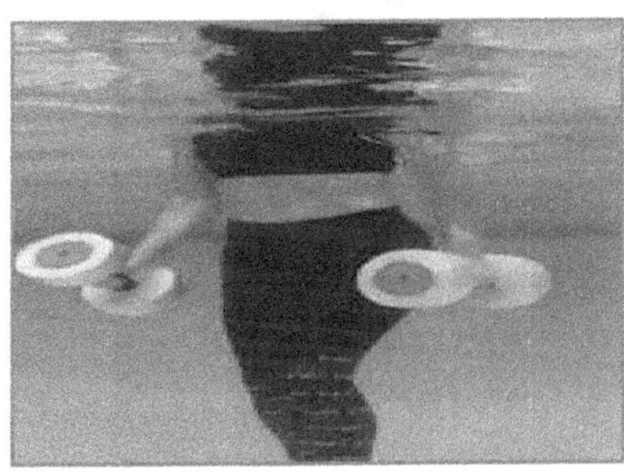
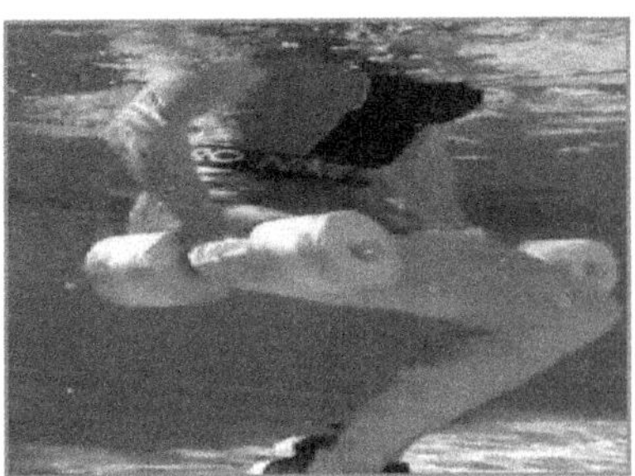

Aqua Zumba

This is a fantastic method to get a cardio exercise while also having fun. Start by imitating the instructor's movements as you follow their lead.

This exercise can be combined with a number of other water aerobics moves.

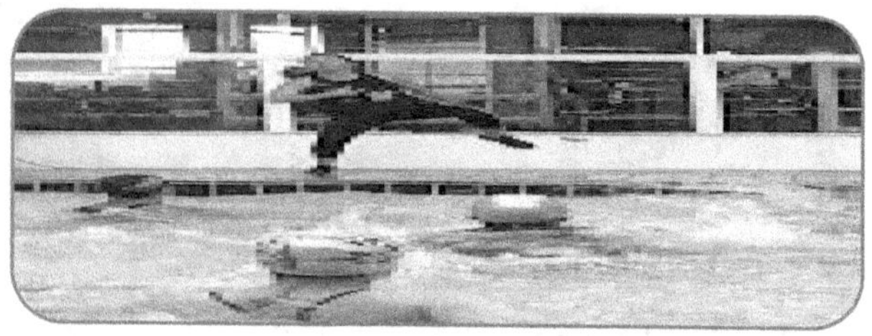

These are only a handful of the numerous water aerobic activities available to you. It's crucial to pick workouts that are effective for your fitness level and will give you a solid workout.

CHAPTER 3: COOL-DOWN EXERCISES

Arm Circles

Your shoulders and arms will be greatly relaxed after doing this. Start by standing in waist-deep water and making broad, forward- and backward-moving circles with your arms. This exercise can also be performed with the arms raised overhead.

Leg Swings

Your legs and hips can be relaxed by doing this. Swing your legs back and forth while standing in waist-deep water with your knees slightly bent. This exercise can also be performed with your legs extended to the sides.

Slow Walking

This is a moderate method for lowering body temperature and assisting with the recovery of a normal heartbeat. Walk slowly at first in the water up to your waist. This workout can also be performed on a water treadmill.

After water aerobics, slowly stroll to unwind.

Stretching

You can increase your flexibility and range of motion by stretching. You can stretch in a variety of ways, but the following are options to try after a session of water aerobics:

Standing Hamstring stretch: One of the simplest stretches to perform is the one-legged standing hamstring stretch:

- Keep your knee straight while standing up straight in waist-deep water with one heel resting on a yoga block or stool.
- Raise both arms so they are almost level with your ears.
- Keep your back upright by raising your arms rather than lowering them toward your foot.
- Slightly arc your hips forward. Your hamstring behind your thigh should feel stretched.
- Repeat three times, holding the stretch for 15 to 30 seconds each time.
- Carry on with the opposite leg.

Quadriceps stretch: This is a low-impact workout that targets stretching the quadriceps muscles, which are found on the front of the legs. By stretching your quads, you can increase your short-term range of motion and lower your risk of quad injury while standing, walking, or climbing.

- The Quadriceps Stretch should be performed as follows:
- Put your weight on your right leg as you stand in water that is about waist deep.
- Grab your left foot with your left hand and raise it off the ground.
- When your quadriceps start to feel stretched, pull your left foot toward your buttocks.
- After holding the stretch for 30 seconds, switch to the other leg and repeat.
- Repeat three times, holding each stretch for 15 to 30 seconds.
- Follow the same procedure with the other leg.

Chest stretch: Chest stretches are healthy activities that help increase the range of motion, and flexibility, and lower the risk of strain or injury to the chest muscles. The pectoralis major and pectoralis minor muscles comprise most of the chest's primary muscular group. To maintain a healthy upper body, stretching the chest should be an integral part of any stretching and exercise regimen.

Here are some chest stretches that work well when performed while standing in approximately waist-deep water:

Chest stretch with two arms: With your arms raised to shoulder height and facing ahead, stand tall with your feet shoulder-width apart. Push your arms back until you feel a stretch in your chest. Hold the stretch for ten to thirty seconds.

Double Arm Stretch Chest with Arms behind Back: Standing tall with your feet shoulder-width apart, lift your arms behind your back, then interlace your fingers with your palms facing each other in a double arm stretch. Till your chest stretches, push your arms back and upward. Hold the space for ten to thirty seconds.

Stretch using Anchor:

Stretching with an Anchor (Wall, Pole, etc.): Place your feet shoulder-width apart and stand 2-3 feet from your anchor point (Wall, Pole). Push your arm straight back until you experience some minor discomfort with one arm raised to the anchor point at shoulder height. After holding the stretch for 10 to 30 seconds, switch arms and repeat.

Elbow Stretch with Arms above Head for Chest:

Standing upright with your feet shoulder-width apart, lock your fingers with your arms behind and above your head to stretch your elbows for your chest. Push your elbows back gradually until your chest begins to expand. For 10 to 20 seconds, hold.

Corner Stretch for Chest:

Standing facing a pool corner, rest your hands on the wall a few feet away from the corner, and lean into the wall until you feel your chest extend. Maintain for 10–30 seconds.

Shoulder stretch: Stretching the shoulders regularly is important for keeping the muscles flexible, avoiding injuries, and easing neck and shoulder pain and tension. The complex shoulder joint is prone to a number of problems, including tendonitis in the rotator cuff, arthritis, and tears. Regular stretching of the shoulder joint's supporting muscles can increase range of motion, lessen pain, and increase safety.

Here are some effective shoulder stretches that could be done in waist-deep water:

Neck Stretch:

Stand with your feet hip-width apart, your arms at your sides, and your gaze forward. Try touching the ear to the shoulder on each side of your head as you slowly tilt it to the right and left. Repeat three times while maintaining the position for 10 seconds on each side.

Shoulder Rolls:

Allow the arms to drop down at your sides as you stand with your feet hip-width apart. When you move your shoulders back, press your shoulder blades together, lift them up toward your ears, and then lower them. To feel the stretch at the back of the shoulders, move the elbows forward. Do this ten times.

Pendulum:

Place your right hand on a table or chair for support while you stand with your feet hip-width apart and lean forward. Allowing gravity to assist the movement, swing the left arm gently in little circular motions while letting it hang down. For another 30 to 60 seconds, repeat the process with the other arm.

Cross-Body Arm Swings:

Standing with your feet hip-width apart, extend your arms out to the sides, and while keeping both arms straight, cross your right arm across your left. Cross the left arm over the right after bringing the arms back out to the sides. Do this ten times.

Cross-Body Shoulder Stretch:

Standing with your feet hip-width apart, pull your right arm across your body with your palm towards the floor on the opposite side of your left leg. Hook the left forearm under the right arm by bending the left arm at the elbow. Stretch the back of the right shoulder by pulling the right arm farther in and across the body with the aid of the left forearm. Continue on the opposite side after holding for 20 seconds.

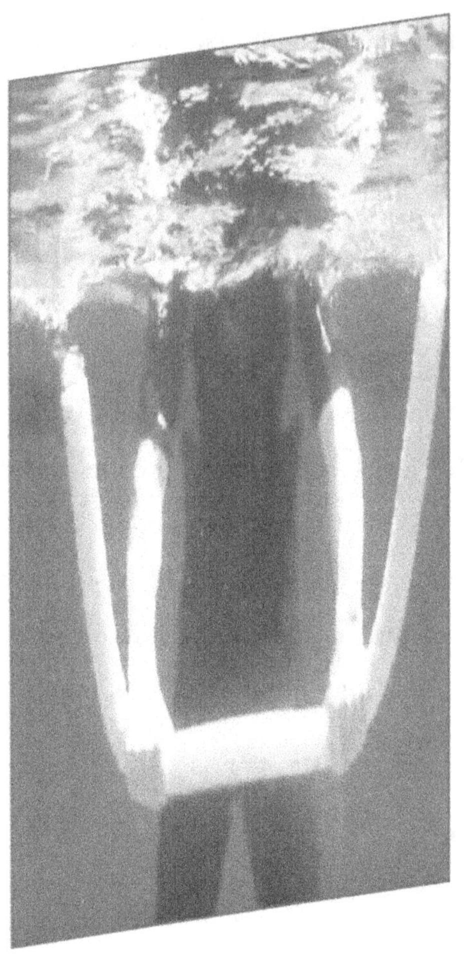

CONCLUSION

Guidelines for Water Aerobics Safety

Although Water Aerobics is a terrific method to work out, this should always be done safely. Here are a few advices:

Begin gradually. If you are new to water aerobics, start out with a short workout and gradually extend your time in the water

Be aware of your body. Be aware of your body. Stop working out and take a break if you start to hurt.

Remain hydrated. Water is important to consume before, during, and after exercise.

Put sunblock on. You can still acquire a sunburn even when you are in the water.

Observe your surroundings carefully. Swim with a partner and watch out for slick places.

Resources

To learn more about water aerobics and how to be safe, there are a lot of resources accessible. To name a few:

- The American Red Cross provides water aerobics sessions and instructor training.

- The Aquatic Exercise Association is a specialized group that supports water aerobics instructors and participants by offering them resources.

- The National Academy of Sports Medicine administers a certification program for instructors of water aerobics.

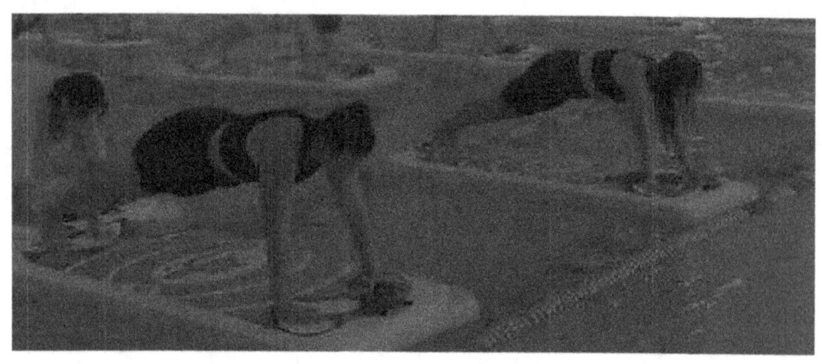

Thank You for Embarking on Your Water Aerobics Journey

Dear reader,

We want to express our heartfelt gratitude for joining us on this exciting journey into the world of water aerobics. Your decision to purchase our book shows your commitment to improving your health, fitness, and overall well-being through the joy of aquatic exercise.

As you flip through the pages and explore the exercises, techniques, and insights we've shared, remember that every step you take in the water is a step towards a healthier you. The soothing embrace of water and the invigorating rhythm of the workouts will not only benefit your body but also your mind and soul.

This book is more than just a guide; it's a companion on your path to wellness. Embrace the gentle resistance of the water, feel the music of movement, and let the waves of energy propel you towards your goals.

Thank you for choosing us as part of your water aerobics journey. We can't wait to hear about your achievements, experiences, and the waves of positivity that this journey brings into your life.

Dive in, stay active, and enjoy every splash of progress!

With heartfelt gratitude,

Robert M.Peery

AEROBICS TRACKER

DAY	WORKOUT TYPE	TIME SPENT	REMARK
Monday			
Tuesday			
Wednesday			
Thursday			
Friday			
Saturday			
Sunday			

AEROBICS TRACKER

DAY	WORKOUT TYPE	TIME SPENT	REMARK
Monday			
Tuesday			
Wednesday			
Thursday			
Friday			
Saturday			
Sunday			

AEROBICS TRACKER

DAY	WORKOUT TYPE	TIME SPENT	REMARK
Monday			
Tuesday			
Wednesday			
Thursday			
Friday			
Saturday			
Sunday			

AEROBICS TRACKER

DAY	WORKOUT TYPE	TIME SPENT	REMARK
Monday			
Tuesday			
Wednesday			
Thursday			
Friday			
Saturday			
Sunday			

AEROBICS TRACKER

DAY	WORKOUT TYPE	TIME SPENT	REMARK
Monday			
Tuesday			
Wednesday			
Thursday			
Friday			
Saturday			
Sunday			

AEROBICS TRACKER

DAY	WORKOUT TYPE	TIME SPENT	REMARK
Monday			
Tuesday			
Wednesday			
Thursday			
Friday			
Saturday			
Sunday			

AEROBICS TRACKER

DAY	WORKOUT TYPE	TIME SPENT	REMARK
Monday			
Tuesday			
Wednesday			
Thursday			
Friday			
Saturday			
Sunday			

AEROBICS TRACKER

DAY	WORKOUT TYPE	TIME SPENT	REMARK
Monday			
Tuesday			
Wednesday			
Thursday			
Friday			
Saturday			
Sunday			

AEROBICS TRACKER

DAY	WORKOUT TYPE	TIME SPENT	REMARK
Monday			
Tuesday			
Wednesday			
Thursday			
Friday			
Saturday			
Sunday			

AEROBICS TRACKER

DAY	WORKOUT TYPE	TIME SPENT	REMARK
Monday			
Tuesday			
Wednesday			
Thursday			
Friday			
Saturday			
Sunday